KIDNEY DISEASE DIET FOR SENIORS ON STAGE 3 FOOD LISTS

Complete Food Lists with GI, potassium, calcium, Sodium, and Phosphorus Values — A Balanced, Healthy Eating Guide for Diabetes and Kidney Disease

Richie Smile Walker

Disclaimer

This publication is designed to provide competent and reliable information regarding the subject covered. However, the views expressed in this publication are those of the author alone, and should not be taken as expert instruction or professional advice. The reader is responsible for his or her actions. The author hereby disclaims any responsibility or liability whatsoever that is incurred from the use or application of the contents of this publication by the purchaser of the reader. The purchaser or reader is hereby responsible for his or her actions.

Table of Contents

Introduction

Hello and welcome to "Kidney Disease Diet for Seniors on Stage 3 Food List." I'm so glad you decided to check out this book, and I'm excited to be your guide on this journey toward better health and well-being.

Let's start by talking about our hardworking kidneys. They often don't get the attention they deserve until something goes wrong. If you or someone you care about is dealing with stage 3 kidney disease, you probably already know how important it is to give these crucial organs some extra care. And you know what? One fantastic way to do that is by following a smart, kidney-friendly diet.

Throughout this book, we'll delve into the world of stage 3 kidney disease, specifically tailored for our beloved seniors. We'll talk about what you should eat and what to avoid, using a friendly, easy-to-understand tone. No complex medical terms or confusing language here—just straightforward, practical advice that you can put into action right away.

Together, we'll learn how to prepare delicious meals that not only support your kidney health but also satisfy your taste buds. We'll uncover the power of specific nutrients and the secrets to maintaining a balanced diet without giving up on flavor. We'll even address tricky situations, like dining out with friends or managing those sudden cravings for foods that aren't quite kidney-friendly.

Whether you're personally dealing with kidney disease or you're a caregiver or family member supporting a loved one through this journey, this book is here to be your reliable guide, your friendly companion, and your source of inspiration. Let's get started, roll up our sleeves, and dive into the world of kidney-friendly cuisine, taking a significant step toward a healthier and happier life.

The Importance of Diet in Managing Kidney Disease for Seniors

Alright, let's talk about why what you eat is so crucial when you're dealing with stage 3 kidney disease. Think of the food you put in your body as the fuel your kidneys need to keep going strong.

When your kidneys aren't feeling their best, they could use a helping hand. And you know what? A well-thought-out diet can be just that. By choosing the right foods and being mindful of what to cut back on, you're giving your kidneys a pat on the back.

But it's not just about your kidneys – it's about keeping your entire body in top shape. You want to maintain your energy levels, keep those nutrients in check, and avoid anything that might strain those hardworking organs.

The great news is, you don't have to settle for boring meals. We'll explore how you can still enjoy your food while taking care of those kidneys. It's all about finding that perfect balance where delicious meets healthy.

So, get ready, because we're about to uncover how your food choices can be your secret weapon in managing stage 3 kidney disease. It's not just about what's on your plate; it's about giving your body the best shot at feeling great. Let's get started!

Understanding Stage 3 Kidney Disease in Seniors:

Let's break down what's going on with stage 3 kidney disease, particularly for our older folks. Picture your kidneys as these super crucial filters in your body. They work hard to keep things in check, but when they hit stage 3, it's like they're not working as smoothly as they used to.

In this stage, things are getting a bit serious. It's not a minor issue, but it's not a major red alert either. It's like a middle ground that needs some extra attention.

For our senior friends, this could mean a bit of a rough ride. You might notice changes in how you feel, like being more tired or less energetic than before. Suddenly, those regular checkups with the doctor become a bit more frequent.

But don't worry! We're here to help you understand what's happening and how you can handle this stage. We'll discuss what to look out for, what signs to keep an eye on, and how to make some adjustments to help you feel as good as possible.

Overview of the Book's Purpose and Structure:

Let me give you the rundown of what this book is all about and how it's set up. The main aim here is to be your reliable guide on the journey to managing stage 3 kidney disease, specially designed for seniors.

We'll start by digging into why your diet is a big player in this scenario. I'll explain how every bite you take can make a real difference in how you feel. Then, we'll take a closer look at what stage 3 kidney disease truly means for you or your loved ones. It's all about understanding what's happening inside and finding the best way to navigate through it.

Next up, we'll get to the good stuff – the diet plan. I'll share some easy-to-follow guidelines on what you should put on your plate and what's better to leave out. But wait, it's not all about restrictions! We'll also talk about how to make your meals tasty and satisfying because, let's face it, we all deserve to enjoy what we eat.

And of course, we'll cover all the little details, like handling meals out or dealing with those sneaky cravings. I want this book to be your go-to resource, your friendly companion, making sure you have all the tools you need to feel your best while managing stage 3 kidney disease.

So get ready to soak up some knowledge, grab some practical tips, and maybe even have a bit of fun along the way. Let's dive in and make this journey as smooth and enjoyable as possible!

Understanding Kidney Disease in Seniors

Explaining the Function of the Kidneys

Let's talk about our hardworking kidneys and what they do for our bodies. You can think of them as these amazing filters that work non-stop to keep our system in balance. They help get rid of waste, extra water, and other stuff we don't need in our blood. But that's not all – they also play a crucial role in keeping our blood pressure in check and making sure our bodies have the right amount of important minerals like sodium, potassium, and phosphorus. They even lend a hand in making red blood cells and activating vitamin D, which keeps our bones strong and our muscles working properly. Knowing all about these incredible jobs the kidneys do gives us a solid foundation for understanding how kidney disease can affect seniors.

Common Causes and Risk Factors for Kidney Disease in Seniors

As we get older, the chances of having kidney problems go up, so it's important to understand what might lead to kidney disease. Things like high blood pressure, diabetes, or having a family history of kidney issues can put seniors at a higher risk. Some everyday choices like eating too much salt or unhealthy fats, smoking, or not being active enough can also take a toll on the kidneys. Even certain health conditions like heart disease or being overweight can play a role in how kidney disease develops in seniors. By knowing about these causes and risks, seniors and their caregivers can take steps to prevent or manage kidney issues before they become more serious.

Symptoms and Complications of Stage 3 Kidney Disease

When the kidneys start having trouble and reach stage 3, seniors might notice some changes in how they feel. Things like feeling extra tired, not being as hungry, having trouble focusing, or experiencing muscle cramps and swelling in the hands and feet can become more noticeable. Seniors with stage 3 kidney disease might also face complications such as anemia, bone problems, imbalances in important body chemicals, and even issues with their heart and blood vessels, all of which can affect their overall well-being. Knowing these symptoms and complications early on helps seniors and their doctors find ways to manage and lessen the effects of stage 3 kidney disease.

Understanding the ins and outs of kidney function, the common causes and risks for kidney disease in seniors, and the symptoms and complications that come with stage 3 kidney disease can give seniors and their caregivers a clearer picture of why following a kidney-friendly diet and lifestyle is so important. This knowledge lays the groundwork for making effective changes to their diet and lifestyle, ultimately improving how seniors manage their stage 3 kidney disease and enhancing their overall quality of life.

The Role of Diet in Managing Kidney Disease

Importance of tailoring a Diet Plan for Seniors with stage 3 Kidney Disease

A customized and well-thought-out nutrition plan is an essential component that may make a huge impact when treating elders with stage 3 renal disease. Let's explore why this customized nutrition plan is a vital component of the toolkit of tactics used to assist elders' health throughout this difficult transition.

The first and most important consideration when creating a diet plan for seniors with stage 3 renal disease is the special nutritional demands resulting from impaired kidney function. This kind of diet makes sure that the foods chosen are easy on the kidneys, which lessens the strain on these important organs and encourages their best possible functioning.

Additionally, a customized meal plan helps support the management and upkeep of the delicate equilibrium of vital nutrients, including potassium, salt, phosphorus, and protein, which are critical for sustaining general health and wellbeing. Customizing the diet to regulate the intake of these nutrients may greatly reduce the likelihood of developing further difficulties and pain related to stage 3 renal disease.

Moreover, a well-designed diet plan provides the chance to achieve a balance between keeping a healthy body weight and guaranteeing a sufficient intake of essential nutrients. For seniors in particular, maintaining this balance is essential because it supports the treatment of various health issues that may coexist with renal disease and helps avoid further burden on the kidneys.

Customizing a diet plan for elderly individuals with stage 3 renal disease is also essential for meeting the unique nutritional needs of this population, including decreased appetite, altered taste preferences, and reduced physical activity. These variables may be taken into consideration using a customized strategy, guaranteeing that the diet stays sustainable and pleasurable for the person while still being kidney-friendly.

All things considered, it is crucial to customize a meal plan for elderly patients with stage 3 renal disease. We can provide seniors the greatest opportunity to successfully manage their disease, improve their quality of life, and advance their general well-being by tailoring their diet to their specific nutritional demands and obstacles.

Impact of Nutrition on Kidney Function for seniors

The importance of diet in helping elders maintain their renal function cannot be emphasized. Their dietary decisions eventually impact their general health and well-being by either strengthening or weakening their kidneys.

First and foremost, seniors may preserve healthy renal function with a diet rich in nutrients and well-balanced. A diet high in vital vitamins and minerals, such as vitamin B6, folate, and antioxidants, together with enough water helps boost the kidneys' capacity to filter waste and maintain fluid balance while also improving overall renal health.

Moreover, seniors with impaired renal function must consume the proper balance of proteins. Maintaining muscle mass and preventing muscle wasting may be achieved with a regulated but sufficient protein diet, which also helps to reduce the amount of waste products the kidneys have to deal with. However, consuming too much protein may strain the kidneys, which may exacerbate existing problems and cause new ones.

In addition, monitoring the consumption of minerals including phosphorus, potassium, and salt is essential for maintaining renal function in older adults. Maintaining fluid balance, preventing the accumulation of dangerous chemicals in the circulation, and controlling the quantities of these minerals in the diet may all help control blood pressure and lessen the burden on the kidneys.

Additionally, a balanced diet that helps elders maintain a healthy body weight may have a substantial influence on renal function. While weight reduction attained by a well-managed diet may lessen the stress on the kidneys and reduce the evolution of the illness, obesity, and overweight can accelerate the advancement of renal disease.

Important Nutrients for Seniors with Chronic Kidney Disease to Consider

Now that we've covered the essentials, let's discuss the foods that you should watch out for if you have a renal illness. The way you feel and how well your kidneys function may both be significantly impacted by these essential minerals.

Let's talk about protein first. This involves a little bit of balance. Make sure you're receiving enough to maintain the health of those muscles but avoid obtaining too much to the point where your kidneys are overworked. Therefore, while choosing your sources of protein, choose quality before quantity.

The next item on the list is to monitor your consumption of salt. Consuming excessive amounts of salt may have negative effects on your health, such as increased blood pressure and increased renal workload. Thus, keep an eye out for those deceptive salt sources that might be found in processed and packaged meals.

Another player to be aware of is potassium. It's a vital mineral that keeps your heart and muscles functioning, but excessive quantities might interfere with your heart's natural rhythm. Thus, be cautious while consuming foods rich in potassium, such as potatoes, bananas, and certain legumes.

Phosphorus is being considered as well. Numerous foods contain it, and while it's necessary for healthy bones and teeth, too much of it might upset your body's mineral balance. Watch out for phosphorus in certain whole grains, dairy products, and nuts.

Last but not least, remember to drink plenty of water. Here, water is your greatest ally. It keeps everything running properly and aids in the kidneys' removal of waste.

The Stage 3 Kidney Disease Diet Plan

General guidelines and principles of the diet for seniors

Crafting a diet plan for seniors, especially those dealing with kidney disease, involves following some helpful guidelines and principles. These guidelines are aimed at promoting overall health and well-being while minimizing the strain on the kidneys, ensuring a better quality of life.

The key is to focus on a well-balanced and nutrient-rich diet. This means including a variety of fresh fruits and vegetables, whole grains, lean proteins, and healthy fats in daily meals. Opting for whole, unprocessed foods while avoiding highly processed and high-sodium options can greatly benefit seniors, as it helps control blood pressure and reduces fluid retention, which impacts kidney function.

Controlling portion sizes is also essential in managing the diet for seniors. Keeping an eye on portion sizes helps regulate the intake of specific nutrients like protein, sodium, and phosphorus, all of which directly affect kidney health. It also aids in weight management, a crucial factor that can influence the progression of kidney disease and impact overall senior health.

Another vital principle is to emphasize the importance of staying hydrated. Encouraging seniors to drink enough fluids, mainly water, is key to supporting proper kidney function and preventing dehydration, which can lead to various health issues. Striking a balance between fluid intake and any fluid restrictions advised by healthcare providers is crucial to prevent the build-up of excess fluid in the body, which can strain the kidneys.

Furthermore, seniors should regularly monitor their nutritional intake and make any necessary adjustments to their meal plans. This personalized approach ensures that the diet plan remains tailored to the individual's specific health needs, ultimately helping seniors manage kidney disease better and supporting their overall well-being.

Recommended Foods for Seniors with Stage 3 Kidney Disease

Here is a list of recommended foods for seniors with stage 3 kidney disease, along with explanations:

1. **Apples:** A delicious low-potassium fruit that provides fiber and supports digestive health. Enjoy them fresh, in salads, or baked for a sweet and healthy treat.

2. **Bell peppers:** These vibrant veggies are low in potassium and rich in immune-boosting nutrients. Use them in salads, stir-fries, or as tasty stuffed peppers.

3. **Cauliflower:** A versatile cruciferous veggie that's low in potassium and high in essential vitamins. Roast it, mash it, or add it to soups and stews for a nutritious twist.

4. **Dried cranberries:** These sweet and tangy treats are low in potassium and packed with fiber and antioxidants. Add them to salads, oatmeal, or baked goods for a flavorful punch.

5. **Eggs:** A protein powerhouse with low potassium levels, perfect for supporting muscle health. Enjoy them boiled, or scrambled, or use them in various recipes for added protein.

6. **Fennel:** This low-potassium vegetable has a unique licorice-like flavor and is rich in vitamins and minerals. Add it to salads, roast it, or use it in soups and stews for a fragrant and nutritious meal.

7. **Grapes:** A hydrating, low-potassium fruit packed with vitamins and antioxidants, promoting heart health. Enjoy them fresh, frozen, or in fruit salads for a sweet and refreshing treat.

8. **Honeydew melon:** This refreshing fruit is low in potassium and provides essential vitamins, perfect for overall health. Enjoy it fresh, in fruit salads, or blended into smoothies for a hydrating and delicious beverage.

9. **Iceberg lettuce:** A hydrating and low-potassium lettuce variety perfect for salads, sandwiches, and wraps. Add it to various recipes for some crunch and a refreshing component.

10. **Jicama:** A crunchy and low-potassium root vegetable that supports digestive health with its dietary fiber and nutrients. Enjoy it as a standalone snack, in salads, or stir-fries for a satisfying crunch and subtle sweetness.

11. **Lemons:** These citrus fruits provide moderate potassium levels and are rich in vitamins and antioxidants, perfect for boosting the immune system. Use them to add a tangy kick to beverages, salads, or marinades.

12. **Mangoes:** A tropical delight with high fiber content and rich in vitamins, benefiting digestive health and immune function. Enjoy them fresh, in fruit salads, or blended into smoothies for a sweet and exotic flavor.

13. **Nectarines:** Low in potassium and high in essential nutrients, these stone fruits are a delicious and

nutritious option for seniors. Enjoy them fresh, in desserts, or savory dishes for a sweet and tangy twist.

14. **Oats:** A whole grain with low potassium levels, rich in dietary fiber, and great for heart health and digestion. Enjoy them as oatmeal, baked goods, or savory recipes for a nourishing meal.

15. **Peas:** These low-potassium legumes are a great source of protein and dietary fiber, supporting muscle health and overall well-being. Add them to soups, stews, or salads for a hearty and nutritious option.

16. **Quinoa:** A low-potassium whole grain packed with essential amino acids and dietary fiber, perfect for promoting overall health and well-being. Use it as a base for salads, a side dish, or in various recipes for added nutrition and texture.

17. **Raspberries:** These antioxidant-rich fruits are low in potassium, making them a kidney-friendly option for seniors. Enjoy them fresh, in desserts, or smoothies for a naturally sweet and tangy flavor.

18. **Strawberries:** Low in potassium and high in vitamins and antioxidants, these are perfect for boosting the immune system. Enjoy them fresh, in salads, or desserts for a naturally sweet and refreshing taste.

19. **Tofu:** A low-potassium, low-sodium protein source, ideal as a meat alternative for seniors. Grill it, bake it, or add it to stir-fries and soups for a versatile and nutritious option.

20. **Udon noodles:** These low-potassium noodles are great for various culinary preparations, providing a versatile base for soups, stir-fries, and salads. Combine them with different ingredients for a satisfying and kidney-friendly meal.

21. **Vinaigrette dressing:** This low-potassium, low-sodium dressing option can enhance the flavor of salads and other dishes. Make it with olive oil, vinegar, and herbs for a light and refreshing addition to meals.

22. **Watermelon (Xigua):** This hydrating fruit is low in potassium and rich in essential vitamins and minerals, perfect for overall health and well-being. Enjoy it fresh, frozen, or blended into beverages for a naturally sweet and refreshing option.

23. **Yogurt:** This low-potassium, low-sodium dairy option provides essential probiotics and nutrients, promoting seniors' digestive health. Enjoy it as a standalone snack, in smoothies, or in various culinary preparations for a creamy and nutritious addition.

24. **Zucchini:** This low-potassium vegetable is a versatile ingredient rich in vitamins and minerals, perfect for seniors' overall health and well-being. Enjoy it roasted, grilled, or in soups and stews for added texture and nutrition.

25. **Asparagus:** A unique and earthy vegetable low in potassium, packed with essential vitamins and minerals. Roast it, grill it, or sauté it as a standalone side dish or use it in various culinary preparations.

26. **Blueberries:** These antioxidant-rich berries are low in potassium, making them a kidney-friendly option for seniors. Enjoy them fresh, in desserts, or smoothies for a naturally sweet and tart flavor.

27. **Cucumber:** A hydrating and low-potassium vegetable that adds a refreshing and crunchy element to various dishes. Slice it and add it to salads, use it as a garnish, or enjoy it as a standalone snack for a cool and hydrating treat.

28. **Dates:** These low-potassium fruits are rich in essential vitamins and minerals, supporting overall health and well-being for seniors. Enjoy them as a naturally sweet snack, in desserts, or in baking for a rich and chewy texture.

29. **Edamame:** These low-potassium legumes offer a great source of protein and dietary fiber, promoting muscle health and overall well-being. Enjoy them as a standalone snack, in salads, or stir-fries and soups.

30. **Figs:** These low-potassium fruits are rich in essential vitamins and dietary fiber, supporting digestive health for seniors. Enjoy them fresh, dried as a naturally sweet treat, or in various culinary preparations for added flavor and nutrition.

31. **Garlic:** A flavorful and low-potassium seasoning option that enhances the taste of various dishes. Use it in soups, stews, and sauces, or roast it with vegetables for added aroma and depth of flavor.

32. **Honey:** This natural and low-potassium sweetener option can add a touch of sweetness to beverages, desserts, and baked goods. Drizzle it over yogurt, add it to tea, or use it in marinades for a naturally sweet and flavorful taste.

33. **Almond milk:** A low-potassium alternative to dairy milk that provides essential vitamins and minerals, offering a nutritious option for seniors. Use it in smoothies, cereal, or coffee as a dairy-free and kidney-friendly substitute.

34. **Bananas:** These low-to-moderate potassium fruits are rich in essential vitamins and minerals, supporting heart health and digestion for seniors. Enjoy them fresh, in smoothies, or in baking for a naturally sweet and filling option.

35. **Cabbage:** A low-potassium cruciferous vegetable that offers essential vitamins and dietary fiber, promoting digestive health and overall well-being for seniors. Use it in salads, coleslaw, or stir-fries for a versatile and nutritious meal option.

36. **Eggplant:** This low-potassium vegetable is a versatile and flavorful ingredient in various recipes, providing essential vitamins and minerals for seniors. Enjoy it grilled, roasted, or in stews and casseroles for added texture and taste.

37. **Flaxseeds:** These low-potassium seeds offer essential omega-3 fatty acids and dietary fiber, promoting heart health and digestive function for seniors. Add them to smoothies, yogurt, or baked goods for a nutty and nutritious boost.

38. **Ginger:** A flavorful and low-potassium spice that offers potential anti-inflammatory and digestive benefits for seniors. Use it in teas, soups, stir-fries, or desserts for a warming and aromatic addition to various dishes.

39. **Icing sugar:** A low-potassium sweetener option that can be used in moderation for preparing desserts and baked goods. Use it to sweeten frosting, glazes, or toppings for a delightful and kidney-friendly treat.

40. **Jerusalem artichoke:** A low-potassium root vegetable that provides essential dietary fiber and nutrients, supporting digestive health for seniors. Roast it, sauté it, or use it in soups and stews for a nutty and flavorful addition to meals.

41. **Kiwi:** These low-to-moderate potassium fruits offer essential vitamins and antioxidants, supporting immune health and overall well-being for seniors. Enjoy them fresh, in fruit salads, or smoothies for a tangy and refreshing taste.

42. **Mint:** A low-potassium herb that adds a refreshing and aromatic flavor to various dishes and beverages. Use it in teas, and salads, or add it to water for a naturally invigorating and kidney-friendly option.

43. **Nutritional yeast:** A low-potassium and dairy-free seasoning option that provides essential vitamins and minerals, offering a savory and cheesy flavor to dishes. Sprinkle it over popcorn, and salads, or use it in recipes for a wholesome and flavorful addition.

44. **Olive oil:** A heart-healthy and low-potassium oil option that provides essential monounsaturated fats and antioxidants, supporting overall well-being for seniors. Use it in dressings, and sautés, or drizzle it over vegetables for a flavorful and nutritious choice.

45. **Papaya:** These low-to-moderate potassium fruits offer essential vitamins and digestive enzymes, promoting digestive health and overall well-being for seniors. Enjoy them fresh, in fruit salads, or blended into smoothies for a naturally sweet and tropical taste.

46. **Quince:** This low-potassium fruit provides essential vitamins and dietary fiber, supporting digestive health for seniors. Use it in desserts, and jams, or add it to savory dishes for a sweet and fragrant flavor.

47. **Radishes:** These low-potassium root vegetables add a crisp and peppery flavor to dishes, providing essential vitamins and minerals for seniors. Enjoy them fresh, in salads, or use them as a garnish for a refreshing and kidney-friendly option.

48. **Sunflower seeds:** These low-potassium seeds offer essential nutrients and antioxidants, supporting heart health and overall well-being for seniors. Enjoy them as a standalone snack, in salads, or use them in baking for a crunchy and nutritious topping.

49. **Tangerines:** These low-to-moderate potassium citrus fruits offer essential vitamins and antioxidants, supporting immune health and overall well-being for seniors. Enjoy them fresh, in salads, or use them in desserts for a naturally sweet and tangy flavor.

50. **Vanilla extract:** This low-potassium flavoring option enhances the taste of various desserts and baked goods. Add it to cakes, cookies, or puddings for a fragrant and kidney-friendly sweet treat.

51. **Walnuts:** These low-potassium nuts offer essential omega-3 fatty acids and antioxidants, supporting heart health and overall well-being for seniors. Enjoy them as a standalone snack, in salads, or use them in baking for a rich and nutty flavor.

52. **Xylitol:** This low-potassium sugar alcohol serves as a sugar substitute in various recipes and beverages. Use it in baking, add it to coffee or tea, or use it to sweeten sauces for a kidney-friendly and sweet taste.

53. **Yellow squash:** This hydrating and low-potassium vegetable provides essential vitamins and minerals, supporting overall health and well-being for seniors. Enjoy it roasted, or grilled, or use it in soups and stews for a mild and versatile option.

54. **Zest:** The flavorful outer part of citrus fruit peel adds a low-potassium and aromatic touch to various dishes and beverages. Add it to marinades, desserts, or salads for a refreshing and kidney-friendly twist.

55. **Anchovies:** These low-potassium fish options offer essential omega-3 fatty acids and protein, supporting heart health and overall well-being for seniors. Use them in salads, pasta dishes, or as a savory topping for a flavorful and nutritious meal.

56. **Basil:** This low-potassium herb adds a fresh and aromatic flavor to various dishes and beverages. Use it in pesto, and salads, or add it to pasta for a fragrant and kidney-friendly culinary addition.

57. **Chia seeds:** These low-potassium seeds provide essential omega-3 fatty acids and dietary fiber, promoting heart health and digestive function for seniors. Add them to smoothies, yogurt, or baked goods for a nutritious and filling option.

58. **Dandelion greens:** These low-potassium leafy greens offer essential vitamins and minerals, supporting digestive health and overall well-being for seniors. Use them in salads, and sautés, or add them to smoothies for a slightly bitter and nutritious option.

59. **Endive:** This low-potassium leafy green adds a slightly bitter and refreshing flavor to various dishes and salads. Use it in salads, or wraps, or serve it as a standalone side dish for a hydrating and kidney-friendly option.

60. **Flounder:** This low-potassium and lean fish option provides essential omega-3 fatty acids and protein, supporting heart health and overall well-being for seniors. Enjoy it grilled, baked, or sautéed for a light and flavorful seafood choice.

61. **Garlic powder:** This low-potassium and flavorful seasoning option enhances the taste of various dishes. Add it to soups, and stews, or use it in marinades for a convenient and kidney-friendly culinary addition.

62. **Hemp seeds:** These low-potassium seeds offer essential omega-3 fatty acids and protein, promoting muscle health and overall well-being for seniors. Add them to smoothies, and salads, or use them in baking for a nutty and nutritious topping.

63. **Iced tea:** This refreshing beverage can be a hydrating and low-potassium option, perfect for seniors looking for a tasty and kidney-friendly drink. Enjoy it plain or with a splash of lemon for added flavor.

64. **Juniper berries:** These low-potassium berries offer a unique and slightly piney flavor to various dishes and beverages. Use them in marinades, and sauces, or add them to meat dishes for a distinctive and kidney-friendly culinary addition.

65. **Kale chips:** These low-potassium snacks are a delicious and nutritious alternative to traditional potato chips. Bake them with a touch of olive oil and seasoning for a crunchy and kidney-friendly treat.

66. **Lemon water:** This hydrating and low-potassium beverage is a simple and refreshing option for seniors. Add a slice of lemon to a glass of water for a naturally flavorful and kidney-friendly drink.

67. **Mushrooms:** These low-potassium fungi offer essential vitamins and minerals, supporting overall health and well-being for seniors. Use them in various recipes for their earthy flavor and versatile culinary potential.

68. **Nutmeg:** This low-potassium spice adds a warm and aromatic touch to various dishes and beverages. Use it in baking, and savory recipes, or add it to beverages for a fragrant and kidney-friendly twist.

69. **Oatmeal cookies:** These low-potassium treats are a delicious and heartwarming snack option for seniors.

Bake them with oats, raisins, and a touch of cinnamon for a kidney-friendly and satisfying indulgence.

70. **Parsley:** This low-potassium herb adds a fresh and vibrant flavor to various dishes and beverages. Use it in salads, sauces, or as a garnish for a flavorful and kidney-friendly culinary addition.

71. **Quail:** This low-potassium and lean poultry option provides essential protein for seniors, supporting muscle health and overall well-being. Roast or grill it for a flavorful and kidney-friendly meat choice.

72. **Rice vinegar:** This low-potassium and tangy vinegar option is a perfect addition to various dressings and sauces. Use it in marinades, salads, or stir-fries for a refreshing and kidney-friendly culinary twist.

73. **Spinach:** This low-potassium leafy green is rich in essential vitamins and minerals, supporting overall health and well-being for seniors. Use it in salads, smoothies, or sautés for a nutrient-packed and kidney-friendly ingredient.

Foods to avoid for Seniors with Stage 3 Kidney Disease

Here is a comprehensive list of foods to avoid for seniors with stage 3 kidney disease, along with explanations:

1. **Avocado:** Avoid this potassium-rich fruit as it can significantly raise potassium levels in the blood, leading to potential issues for those with compromised kidneys.

2. **Beets:** These root vegetables are high in oxalate, which can contribute to kidney stone formation. It's best to steer clear to prevent potential kidney-related problems.

3. **Chocolate:** Skip this sweet treat as it contains high levels of phosphorus, which can complicate matters for seniors with impaired kidney function.

4. **Dried fruits:** These snacks pack a potassium punch that can be harmful to seniors with compromised kidney function. It's best to avoid them.

5. **Excessive salt:** Say no to high-sodium foods as they can raise blood pressure and lead to fluid retention, straining the kidneys.

6. **Fast food:** Steer clear of these high-sodium and high-fat meals as they can exacerbate issues related to blood pressure and fluid retention, especially for seniors with compromised kidneys.

7. **Grapefruit:** This citrus fruit is loaded with potassium, which can spell trouble for individuals with compromised kidney function. It's best to avoid it.

8. **High-phosphorus foods:** Cut back on processed meats, cheese, and whole grains as they are high in phosphorus, which can lead to phosphorus retention and complicate matters for those with impaired kidneys.

9. **Instant noodles:** These convenient foods often come with a sodium overload, which can lead to complications related to blood pressure and fluid retention, straining the kidneys.

10. **Jerky:** Avoid this protein-rich snack as it is high in sodium and can worsen problems related to blood pressure and fluid retention, particularly for seniors with compromised kidneys.

11. **Kale:** This nutritious leafy green is rich in potassium, which can pose challenges for individuals with stage 3 kidney disease. It's best to avoid it.

12. **Lentils:** These legumes are high in phosphorus and can pose challenges for seniors with compromised kidney function. It's better to limit their intake.

13. **Miso soup:** This traditional Japanese soup often contains high levels of sodium, which can strain the kidneys. It's best to skip it to avoid potential complications.

14. **Nuts and seeds:** These snacks are high in phosphorus and can lead to complications for seniors with stage 3 kidney disease. It's best to keep them off the menu.

15. **Organ meats:** The liver and kidney, in particular, are high in phosphorus and can contribute to phosphorus retention. It's best to avoid them to prevent complications.

16. **Packaged snacks:** These often come with a high sodium content, which can lead to complications related to blood pressure and fluid retention, straining the kidneys.

17. **Ramen:** This popular noodle dish often contains high levels of sodium, which can strain the kidneys. It's best to avoid it to prevent potential complications.

18. **Soy sauce:** This condiment is high in sodium and can lead to complications related to blood pressure and fluid retention, especially for seniors with compromised kidneys.

19. **Tomato products:** Tomato sauce and paste are high in potassium, which can be detrimental for individuals with compromised kidney function. It's best to avoid them.

20. **Unregulated herbal supplements:** It's best to avoid these supplements as they can potentially interact with medications and worsen kidney-related complications.

21. **Vitamin C supplements:** Excessive intake of vitamin C supplements can contribute to the formation of kidney stones and other kidney-related issues.

22. **White bread:** This refined grain product can raise blood sugar levels and may pose challenges for seniors with impaired kidney function. It's best to opt for healthier alternatives.

23. **Xanthan gum:** This food additive can potentially lead to gastrointestinal discomfort and may worsen kidney-related complications in some individuals.

24. **Yeast extract:** This flavoring is high in sodium and can lead to complications related to blood pressure and fluid retention, particularly for seniors with compromised kidneys.

25. **Zucchini bread:** This baked good often contains added phosphorus, which can be detrimental for seniors with compromised kidney function. It's best to avoid it to prevent potential complications.

Creating Balanced Meal Plans and Portion Control Strategies

Developing balanced meal planning and putting portion management techniques into practice is crucial to maintaining a healthy diet. This is a thorough instruction on how to prepare meals that are balanced and use sensible portion management techniques:

Understanding Macronutrients: Let's start by talking about the three main macronutrients: lipids, proteins, and carbs. Make sure the body gets a variety of vital nutrients by including a balance of these nutrients in every meal.

Place an Emphasis on entire Foods: Choose entire foods including fruits, vegetables, whole grains, lean meats, and good fats. These options support general health and wellbeing since they are high in dietary fiber, vitamins, and minerals.

Limit Processed Foods: Cut down on the amount of processed foods you eat, since they are usually heavy in sugar, salt, and bad fats. These products may be linked to several health problems, such as weight gain and elevated blood pressure.

Reduce Portion Sizes: To reduce portion sizes and stop overindulging, use measurement instruments. Being aware of serving sizes helps in controlling caloric intake, which is essential for maintaining a healthy weight and avoiding issues brought on by consuming too many nutrients.

Select fewer Plates: To provide the appearance of a bigger plate while eating fewer servings, use smaller plates and bowls. This mental ploy may assist in managing the quantity of food eaten at each meal.

Incorporate Nutrient-Dense Foods: Give priority to foods high in nutrients that provide vital vitamins and minerals without being too caloric. These foods, which promote a variety of physiological processes and general wellbeing, include leafy greens, whole grains, lean proteins, and healthy fats.

Plan Your Meals Ahead of Time: Arrange your meals ahead of time to guarantee that they are balanced in terms of nutrition. Making a weekly meal plan helps facilitate portion management and organization, which will make it simpler to stick to a nutritious and well-balanced diet.

Eat consciously and deliberately, enjoying each meal, and being aware of your body's signals of hunger and fullness. Eating mindfully may help you avoid overindulging and strengthen your relationship with your body's natural hunger and satiety cues.

The Best Foods to Eat for Better Blood Glucose Control

41

Non-Starchy Vegetables:

When it comes to managing blood glucose levels, incorporating non-starchy vegetables like spinach, broccoli, and cauliflower can be highly beneficial. Spinach is packed with essential vitamins and minerals, while broccoli provides fiber and antioxidants. Cauliflower, on the other hand, is a versatile vegetable that can be included in various dishes to help stabilize blood sugar levels.

Whole Grains:

Whole grains such as oatmeal, quinoa, and brown rice can contribute significantly to better blood glucose control. Oatmeal, rich in soluble fiber, can regulate blood sugar levels and improve heart health, while quinoa, a nutrient-dense whole grain, offers a good source of protein and fiber. Brown rice, with its lower glycemic index compared to white rice, serves as a complex carbohydrate that helps stabilize blood sugar levels when consumed in moderation.

Lean Proteins:

Incorporating lean proteins like chicken breast, fish, and tofu can help regulate blood sugar levels and support muscle health. Chicken breast is a versatile and lean protein option that can be prepared in various ways. Fish, particularly salmon and tuna, rich in omega-3 fatty acids, can contribute to improved insulin sensitivity and better blood glucose control. Tofu, a low-fat plant-based protein source, is suitable for individuals following vegetarian or vegan diets.

Healthy Fats:

Including sources of healthy fats such as avocados, nuts, and olive oil in the diet can aid in managing blood glucose levels. Avocados, rich in monounsaturated fats, provide essential nutrients and can improve insulin sensitivity when consumed in moderation. Nuts like almonds and walnuts are packed with healthy fats that can lower blood sugar levels and reduce the risk of developing type 2 diabetes. Olive oil, a key component of the Mediterranean diet, contains monounsaturated fats and antioxidants that contribute to better blood glucose control and heart health.

Legumes:

Legumes such as lentils, beans, and chickpeas are valuable additions to a diabetic-friendly diet. Lentils, high in fiber and protein, have a minimal impact on blood glucose levels and can improve insulin sensitivity. Beans like black beans and kidney beans, packed with fiber and nutrients, have a low glycemic index and help stabilize blood sugar levels when included as part of a balanced meal plan. Chickpeas, a versatile legume, are rich in fiber and protein, supporting better blood glucose control and overall health.

The Worst Foods to Eat for Diabetes

Refined Carbohydrates:

It's essential to avoid refined carbohydrates such as white bread, pasta, and sweetened breakfast cereals as they can cause rapid spikes in blood sugar levels.

Sugary Beverages:

Steer clear of sugary beverages like soda and fruit juices, as they can lead to elevated blood sugar levels and increased risk of insulin resistance.

Processed Meats:

Limit the consumption of processed meats such as sausages and bacon due to their high sodium and unhealthy fat content, which can impact blood sugar control.

High-Sugar Snacks:

Foods like cakes, pastries, cookies, and other high-sugar snacks can cause significant fluctuations in blood glucose levels and should be avoided or consumed in moderation.

Fried Foods:

French fries and fried chicken, high in unhealthy fats, should be avoided to prevent increased insulin resistance and potential risks associated with elevated cholesterol levels.

High-Sodium Foods:

Avoid canned soups and packaged snack foods, as they are high in sodium and unhealthy fats, which can contribute to increased blood pressure and potential complications for individuals with diabetes.

Sugary Desserts:

Limit the intake of sugary desserts like ice cream, puddings, and custards, as they can lead to significant blood sugar spikes and contribute to poor blood sugar control and potential weight gain.

The Potassium, Sodium, and Phosphorus Counter

The Potassium Counter

Seniors with Stage 3 renal disease must be aware of the potassium levels of different meal groups. Potassium is an essential element for healthy neuron and muscle function, but too much of it may be problematic for those with impaired renal function. This chapter will explore the nuances of the potassium counter with an emphasis on certain food groups that are often included in elderly citizens' diets. This chapter attempts to provide readers with the information and resources required for efficient dietary management in the setting of renal illness by offering a thorough examination of each food group.

- **Baked Foods:** Potassium levels in baked products may fluctuate and affect general health, particularly in those who have renal disease. Popular baked goods including bread, cakes, and pastries will be discussed in this section along with their potassium level and useful suggestions for incorporating them into a kidney-friendly diet. It will also showcase substitute products and baking techniques that can lower potassium consumption without sacrificing taste or texture.

- **Beans and Lentils:** Although beans and lentils are well known for their nutritious value, those with renal impairment may find it difficult to process the high potassium concentration in them. In-depth reviews of a variety of beans and lentils will be covered in this part, along with information on potassium content and serving recommendations for seniors with Stage 3 renal disease. It will also highlight innovative cooking methods that optimize the nutritious content of these legumes while reducing potassium consumption.

- **Beverages:** For seniors with Stage 3 renal illness, knowing how much potassium is in various drinks is essential to eating a well-balanced diet. This section will provide a thorough analysis of popular beverage alternatives, including teas, carbonated drinks, and fruit juices, explaining their potassium content and providing advice on how to choose them to promote kidney health. It will stress how crucial it is to keep an eye on how much alcohol you consume and choose low-potassium substitutes to preserve the right mineral balance.

- **Breakfast Cereals:** Breakfast cereals are a common option for many people in the morning, although there may be large variations in their potassium levels. This section will explore the world of morning cereals, evaluating the potassium content and suggesting serving amounts that are appropriate for seniors with renal disease. Additionally, it will provide helpful advice on how to choose low-potassium foods and combine them into a well-balanced meal plan that is customized to meet the dietary requirements of people with Stage 3 renal disease.

- **Dairy and Alternatives:** Although dairy products and their substitutes are valuable providers of vital nutrients, those with impaired renal function may experience negative effects from their high potassium concentration. This section will provide a thorough analysis of several dairy and non-dairy substitutes, highlighting their potassium content and suggesting portion proportions that are suitable for seniors with Stage 3 renal disease. Additionally, it will provide suggestions for choosing dairy alternatives with reduced potassium that nonetheless have nutritional value and promote kidney health.

- **Dressing, Fat, and Oils:** Although oils, fats, and dressings are essential to many culinary preparations, people with renal disease may find that their potassium concentration affects how their diet is managed overall. Insightful evaluations of various dressings, fats, and oils will be presented in this part, along with information on potassium levels and recommendations for older citizens with Stage 3 renal disease. It will stress how crucial it is to promote kidney health by using low-potassium substitutes and thoughtfully including them in meal preparation.

- **Fast Food Products:** The potassium content of fast food products varies widely, which might have an impact on the total potassium consumption of those with impaired renal function. This section will examine common fast food alternatives, highlighting the potassium amount of each item and providing helpful tips for choosing healthier selections. Additionally, it will stress how crucial it is for seniors with Stage 3 renal disease to limit their intake of fast food and choose low-potassium options to improve their kidney health.

- **Fruits and Fruit Products:** Fruits are well known for their nutritional value, however seniors with Stage 3 renal disease may need to take particular caution because of their potassium level. This section will examine a variety of fruits and fruit products, including comprehensive information on their potassium content as well as serving recommendations that are suitable for those with renal disease. In addition, it will provide inventive ways to use low-potassium fruits in meals and snacks, guaranteeing a balanced and kidney-friendly diet.

- **Seafood and Fish:** Seafood and fish are excellent providers of vital minerals, however, their potassium levels might differ. This section will provide a thorough examination of many fish and shellfish varieties, revealing information about their potassium content and emphasizing the need for portion management for elderly patients with Stage 3 renal disease. Additionally, it will provide suggestions for cooking low-potassium fish and shellfish selections in a manner that preserves their nutritional content and promotes kidney health.

- **Pasta and Grains:** Although pasta and grains are common diet staples, those with renal impairment may have concerns due to their high potassium level. This section will look at a variety of grains and pasta alternatives, giving specific information on how much potassium they contain and suggesting portion amounts for a diet that is kidney-conscious. Additionally, it will provide helpful advice on how to choose low-potassium pasta and grains and include them in a well-balanced diet that is specifically designed to meet the nutritional requirements of elderly patients with Stage 3 renal disease.

- **Meats:** Although meats are important sources of protein and minerals, kidney-conscious diets may need to take special care due to their high potassium level. This section will examine different cuts of meat, providing a thorough breakdown of their potassium content and stressing the need for portion management for those with Stage 3 renal disease. Additionally, it will provide suggestions for choosing meat sources low in potassium and cooking them in ways that maintain their nutritional content and promote kidney health.

- **Seeds and Nuts:** Nuts and seeds are high in nutrients and have many health advantages, however those with renal problems may need to be cautious when consuming them due to their potassium concentration. This section will discuss several kinds of nuts and seeds, including information on how much potassium they contain and recommendations for serving amounts that are suitable for seniors with Stage 3 renal disease. To support improved kidney health, it will also provide suggestions for choosing low-potassium nuts and seeds and integrating them into meals and snacks.

- **Herbs and Spices:** Herbs and spices are necessary to provide taste to a variety of recipes, but their potassium concentration may lead to an increased consumption of potassium. This section will cover a wide range of spices and herbs, illuminating their potassium contents and offering recommendations for low-potassium foods for those with Stage 3 renal illness. It will also provide helpful guidance on how to use herbs and spices sensibly to make tasty foods that retain culinary diversity and promote renal health.

- **Vegetables and Vegetable Products:** Although vegetables are essential parts of a balanced diet, people with renal impairment should choose their vegetables carefully and monitor their portion sizes since they might vary in potassium concentration. In-depth information on potassium levels in a variety of vegetables and vegetable products will be covered in this section, along with suggestions for serving amounts that are suitable for seniors with Stage 3 renal disease. Additionally, it will provide helpful advice on how to choose low-potassium vegetables and include them in meals to guarantee a balanced and kidney-friendly diet.

The Counter for Sodium

Understanding the salt concentration of different food groups is critical for seniors with Stage 3 renal disease. Sodium, a mineral necessary for fluid balance and neuronal function, may be problematic when eaten in excess by those with impaired renal function. This chapter will give a complete examination of the salt concentration in several food categories that are typically seen in senior diets.

- **Baked Delights:** Various amounts of salt included in baked products may hurt one's general health, particularly for those who have renal disease. Popular baked goods including bread, cakes, and pastries will be examined in this section along with their salt level and useful suggestions for incorporating them into a kidney-friendly diet. It will also showcase substitute products and baking techniques that assist in lowering salt consumption without sacrificing taste or texture.
- **Lentils with Beans:** Although beans and lentils are well known for their nutritious value, people with renal

impairment may find it difficult to process the high salt content of these foods. In-depth reviews of a variety of beans and lentils will be covered in this part, along with information on salt content and serving recommendations for seniors with Stage 3 renal disease. It will also demonstrate how to prepare beans to retain their nutritious benefits while reducing salt consumption.

- **Beverages:** Seniors with Stage 3 renal disease must keep a well-balanced diet and be aware of the salt levels of various drinks. This section will provide a thorough analysis of popular beverage alternatives, including teas, carbonated drinks, and fruit juices, explaining their salt content and providing advice on how to choose them to promote renal health. It will stress how crucial it is to keep an eye on how much alcohol you consume and choose low-sodium substitutes to preserve the right mineral balance.

- **Cereals for Breakfast:** Breakfast cereals are a common option for many people in the morning, but there may be a large variation in their salt level. An in-depth discussion of breakfast cereals, salt content analysis, and recommended serving sizes for seniors with renal disease will be covered in this episode.

Additionally, it will provide helpful advice on how to choose low-sodium foods and combine them into a well-balanced meal plan that is customized to meet the dietary requirements of those with Stage 3 renal disease.

- **Dairy and Alternatives:** While dairy products and their substitutes are valuable providers of vital nutrients, those with impaired renal function may be affected by their high salt levels. This section will provide a thorough analysis of several dairy and non-dairy substitutes, highlighting the salt content of each and suggesting portion proportions that are suitable for seniors with Stage 3 renal disease. Additionally, it will provide suggestions for choosing dairy alternatives with less salt that nevertheless have nutritional value and promote kidney health.

- **Oils, Fats, and Dressings:** Although oils, fats, and dressings are essential to many culinary preparations, people with renal disease may find it difficult to regulate their diets overall due to the high salt level of these ingredients. This chapter will provide a thoughtful examination of various oils, fats, and dressings, emphasizing their salt content and recommending good choices for elderly patients with

Stage 3 renal disease. It will stress how crucial it is to promote kidney health by using low-sodium substitutes and carefully integrating them into meal preparation.

- **Fast Food:** Fast food products often have different amounts of sodium, which might influence how much salt a person with impaired renal function consumes overall. Popular fast food alternatives will be examined in this area, along with information on how much salt they contain and helpful tips for choosing healthier options. It will also stress how crucial it is for seniors with Stage 3 renal disease to limit their intake of fast food and choose low-sodium substitutes to improve their kidney health.

- **Fruits and their derivatives:** Although fruits are well known for their nutritional value, seniors with Stage 3 renal disease may need to be particularly mindful of their salt intake. This section will examine a variety of fruits and fruit products, including thorough analyses of their salt content as well as recommendations for serving sizes that are suitable for those with renal disease. In addition, it will provide inventive ways to use fruits low in salt in meals and snacks, guaranteeing a balanced and kidney-friendly diet.

- **Seafood and Fish:** Seafood and fish are excellent providers of vital nutrients, however, their salt level varies. This section will provide a thorough examination of various fish and seafood varieties, shedding light on their salt content and emphasizing the need for portion management for elderly individuals with Stage 3 renal disease. It will also provide suggestions on how to choose shellfish and fish that are low in salt and preserve their nutritional content while promoting renal health.

- **Pasta and Grains:** Although pasta and grains are common diet staples, those with renal impairment may have concerns due to their high salt level. This section will look at a variety of grains and pasta alternatives, giving specifics on how much salt they contain and suggesting portion amounts for a diet that is kidney-conscious. Additionally, it will provide helpful advice on how to choose low-sodium pasta and grains and include them in a well-balanced diet that is specifically designed to meet the nutritional requirements of elderly patients with Stage 3 renal disease.

- **Meats:** Meats are important sources of protein and minerals, but in a diet that is kidney-conscious, their salt concentration may need to be carefully considered.

This episode will explore several kinds of meats, providing a thorough examination of their salt content and stressing the need to control portion sizes for those with Stage 3 renal disease. Additionally, it will provide suggestions for choosing meat alternatives low in salt and cooking them in ways that maintain their nutritional content and promote kidney function.

- **Seeds and Nuts:** Nuts and seeds are nutrient-dense snacks with many health advantages, however those with renal disease may need to be cautious when consuming them due to their high salt level. This section will examine several varieties of nuts and seeds, revealing information about their salt content and recommending serving amounts for seniors with Stage 3 renal disease. To support improved kidney health, it will also provide suggestions for choosing low-sodium nuts and seeds and integrating them into meals and snacks.

- **Herbs and Spices:** Herbs and spices are necessary to provide flavor to a variety of recipes, but their high salt level may lead to an excess of sodium consumption. This section will cover a wide range of spices and herbs, illuminating their salt content and offering recommendations for low-sodium foods for those with

Stage 3 renal disease. It will also provide helpful guidance on how to use herbs and spices sensibly to make tasty foods that retain culinary diversity and promote renal health.

- **Produced from vegetables and/or plants:** Vegetables are essential parts of a balanced diet, but since they may vary in salt content, people with renal impairment should choose their vegetables carefully and watch their portion sizes. This section will cover a wide variety of vegetables and vegetable products, offering in-depth analyses of their salt content and suggesting sensible serving sizes for elderly patients with Stage 3 renal disease. Additionally, it will provide helpful advice on how to choose low-sodium veggies and include them in meals to guarantee a balanced and kidney-friendly diet.

The Phosphorus Counter

Considering the phosphorus content of various food categories is crucial for seniors with Stage 3 kidney disease. When people with compromised kidney function consume too much phosphorus, a mineral crucial for bone health and a range of physiological processes, it may be dangerous. This chapter will provide a detailed study of the phosphorus content of numerous food groups often seen in senior diets.

- **Baked Foods:** The different amounts of phosphorus included in baked products may affect one's general health, particularly for those who have renal disease. Popular baked goods including bread, cakes, and pastries will be examined in this section along with their phosphorus level and useful suggestions for incorporating them into a kidney-friendly diet. Additionally, it will showcase substitute products and baking techniques that assist lower phosphorus consumption without sacrificing taste or texture.

- **Lentils with Beans:** Although beans and lentils are well known for their nutritional value, those with renal impairment may find it difficult to digest their high phosphorus level. This section will provide a thorough examination of several kinds of beans and lentils, providing information on their phosphorus content and recommending serving amounts that are suitable for elderly patients with Stage 3 renal disease. It will also demonstrate how to prepare beans to retain their nutritious value while reducing phosphorus consumption.

- **Beverages:** Seniors with Stage 3 renal disease must understand the phosphorus content of various to maintain a well-balanced diet. This section will provide a thorough analysis of popular beverage alternatives, including teas, carbonated drinks, and fruit juices, explaining their phosphorus content and providing advice on how to choose them to promote kidney health. It will stress how crucial it is to keep an eye on how much alcohol you consume and choose low-phosphorus sub to preserve the right mineral balance.

- **Cereals for Breakfast:** Many people choose breakfast cereals in the morning, however, there might be substantial differences in the amount of phosphorus in them. This section will explore the world of morning cereals, evaluating the phosphorus content and suggesting serving amounts that are appropriate for seniors with renal disease. Additionally, it will provide helpful advice on how to choose low-phosphorus foods and include them in a well-balanced meal plan that is customized to meet the dietary requirements of those with Stage 3 renal disease.

- **Dairy and Alternatives:** While dairy products and their substitutes are valuable providers of vital nutrients, those with impaired renal function may be affected by their high phosphorus levels. This section will provide a thorough analysis of several dairy and non-dairy substitutes, highlighting their phosphorus content and suggesting sensible serving amounts for elderly individuals with Stage 3 renal disease. Additionally, it will provide suggestions for choosing dairy alternatives with minimal phosphorus that preserve nutritional value and promote kidney health.

- **Oils, Fats, and Dressings:** While oils, fats, and dressings are essential to many culinary preparations, their phosphorus concentration may affect how well people with renal disease manage their diets overall. Insightful evaluations of various dressings, fats, and oils will be presented in this part, along with information on their phosphorus content and recommendations for elderly citizens with Stage 3 renal disease. It will stress how crucial it is to promote kidney health by using low-phosphorus substitutes and thoughtfully including them in meal preparation.

- **Quick Food Items:** Fast food products often include different amounts of phosphorus, which might have an impact on those with impaired renal function's total phosphorus consumption. To shed light on the phosphorus content of popular fast food selections, this section will assess them and provide helpful tips for choosing healthier choices. Additionally, it will stress how crucial it is for seniors with Stage 3 renal disease to limit their intake of fast food and choose low-phosphorus options to improve their kidney health.

- **Fruits and their derivatives:** While fruits are well known for their nutritional value, seniors with Stage 3 renal disease may want to take particular note of their phosphorus concentration. This section will examine a variety of fruits and fruit products, including comprehensive analyses of their phosphorus content as well as recommendations for serving sizes that are suitable for people with renal disease. In addition, it will provide inventive ways to include fruits low in phosphorus in meals and snacks, guaranteeing a balanced and kidney-friendly diet.

- **Seafood and Fish:** Although they might contain varying amounts of phosphorus, fish, and seafood are excellent suppliers of vital nutrients. This section will provide a thorough examination of various fish and seafood varieties, revealing information about their phosphorus content and emphasizing the need for portion management for elderly individuals suffering from Stage 3 renal disease. Additionally, it will include suggestions for cooking low-phosphorus fish and shellfish in ways that preserve their nutritional content and promote kidney health.

- **Pasta and Grains:** Although pasta and grains are common diet staples, those with renal impairment may have concerns due to their high phosphorus level. This section will look at a variety of grains and pasta alternatives, giving specific details on how much phosphorus they contain and suggesting portion amounts for a diet that is kidney-conscious. Additionally, it will provide helpful advice on how to choose low-phosphorus pasta and grains and include them in a well-balanced diet that is specifically designed to meet the nutritional requirements of elderly patients with Stage 3 renal disease.

- **Meats:** Although meats are important sources of protein and minerals, kidney-conscious diets may need to take special care due to their high phosphorus level. This section will examine different cuts of meat, providing a thorough breakdown of their phosphorus content and stressing the need for portion management for those with Stage 3 renal disease. Additionally, it will provide suggestions for choosing meat sources low in phosphorus and cooking them in ways that maintain their nutritional content and promote kidney health.

- **Seeds and Nuts:** Nuts and seeds are high in nutrients and have many health advantages; nevertheless, those with renal disease may need to be cautious while consuming them due to their high phosphorus level. This section will examine several nut and seed varieties, revealing information about their phosphorus content and recommending serving amounts for seniors with Stage 3 renal disease. To support improved kidney function, it will also provide suggestions for choosing low-phosphorus nuts and seeds and integrating them into meals and snacks.

- **Herbs and Spices:** Herbs and spices are necessary to provide taste to a variety of recipes, but their phosphorus level may lead to an increased consumption of phosphorus. This section will cover a wide range of spices and herbs, elucidating their phosphorus content and offering recommendations for low-phosphorus foods for those with Stage 3 renal disease. It will also provide helpful guidance on how to use herbs and spices sensibly to make tasty foods that retain culinary diversity and promote renal health.

- **Vegetables and Vegetable Products:** Vegetables are essential parts of a balanced diet, but since they might differ in phosphorus content, people with renal disease need to choose them carefully and monitor their portion sizes. This section will cover a wide variety of vegetables and vegetable products, offering in-depth analyses of their phosphorus content and suggesting sensible serving sizes for elderly patients with Stage 3 renal disease. Additionally, it will provide helpful advice on how to choose low-phosphorus vegetables and include them in meals to guarantee a balanced and kidney-friendly diet.

Meal Plan for Seniors with Stage 3 Kidney Disease

Day 1:

- Breakfast: Oatmeal with sliced strawberries and chia seeds.
- Lunch: Lentil soup with a slice of whole-grain bread.
- Dinner: Grilled chicken breast with steamed green beans and quinoa.

Day 2:

- Breakfast: Scrambled eggs with spinach and diced tomatoes, served with whole-grain toast.
- Lunch: Mixed green salad with grilled shrimp and a light vinaigrette dressing.
- Dinner: Baked cod with lemon and herbs, alongside roasted asparagus and brown rice.

Day 3:

- Breakfast: Greek yogurt with blueberries, honey, and chopped almonds.
- Lunch: Chickpea salad with cucumbers, bell peppers, and a lemon-tahini dressing.
- Dinner: Baked turkey meatballs with marinara sauce, zucchini noodles, and a side salad.

Day 4:

- Breakfast: Whole-grain waffles with peaches and low-fat cottage cheese.
- Lunch: Minestrone with kidney beans and vegetables, paired with whole-grain bread.
- Dinner: Grilled salmon with dill, served with sautéed spinach and quinoa.

Day 5:

- Breakfast: Spinach and banana smoothie with ground flaxseeds.
- Lunch: Black bean and corn salad with bell peppers, red onions, and lime dressing.
- Dinner: Stir-fried tofu with broccoli and brown rice.

Day 6:

- Breakfast: Cottage cheese with mango and sunflower seeds.
- Lunch: Quinoa salad with tomatoes, cucumbers, and a lemon-herb dressing.
- Dinner: Baked chicken breast with paprika, alongside steamed carrots and wild rice.

Day 7:

- Breakfast: Poached eggs, sautéed spinach, and whole-grain toast.
- Lunch: Spinach and kale salad with grilled chicken, cherry tomatoes, and balsamic vinaigrette.
- Dinner: Grilled halibut with lemon and herbs, served with roasted Brussels sprouts and quinoa.

Day 8:

- Breakfast: Whole-grain pancakes with bananas and sugar-free syrup.
- Lunch: Tomato and white bean soup, with a side of whole-grain bread.
- Dinner: Grilled shrimp skewers with mixed vegetables and brown rice.

Day 9:

- Breakfast: Yogurt parfait with strawberries, blueberries, and granola.
- Lunch: Tuna salad with mixed greens, cucumbers, and a light vinaigrette dressing.
- Dinner: Baked lean pork chops with steamed asparagus and quinoa.

Day 10:

- Breakfast: Vegetable omelet with bell peppers, onions, and low-fat cheese, served with whole-grain toast.
- Lunch: Lentil and vegetable stew with a slice of whole-grain bread.
- Dinner: Grilled chicken kabobs with bell peppers, onions, and wild rice.

Day 11:

- Breakfast: Mixed berry smoothie bowl with spinach and pumpkin seeds.
- Lunch: Chickpea and vegetable curry with brown rice.
- Dinner: Baked white fish with lemon-herb marinade, roasted cauliflower, and quinoa.

Day 12:

- Breakfast: Pineapple and cottage cheese with chopped walnuts.
- Lunch: Black bean and sweet potato chili, with a side of whole-grain bread.
- Dinner: Grilled turkey breast with roasted sweet potatoes and steamed green beans.

Day 13:

- Breakfast: Whole-grain waffles with mixed berries and low-fat yogurt.
- Lunch: Spinach salad with grilled shrimp, tomatoes, and a light vinaigrette dressing.
- Dinner: Stir-fried tofu with mixed vegetables and brown rice.

Day 14:

- Breakfast: Scrambled eggs with sautéed mushrooms and whole-grain toast.
- Lunch: Minestrone with kidney beans and vegetables, served with whole-grain bread.
- Dinner: Baked salmon with lemon-dill sauce, roasted Brussels sprouts, and quinoa.

Day 15:

- Breakfast: Overnight oats with peaches and chia seeds.
- Lunch: Quinoa salad with mixed vegetables and lemon vinaigrette.
- Dinner: Baked cod with sautéed broccoli and wild rice.

Day 16:

- Breakfast: Avocado toast with a poached egg.
- Lunch: Lentil and vegetable stew with a side of quinoa.

- Dinner: Grilled chicken breast with balsamic glaze, roasted sweet potatoes, and steamed broccoli.

Day 17:

- Breakfast: Mixed fruit salad with Greek yogurt and chia seeds.
- Lunch: Vegetable and white bean soup with whole-grain bread.
- Dinner: Baked cod with lemon-herb seasoning, sautéed green beans, and wild rice.

Day 18:

- Breakfast: Whole-grain pancakes with bananas and maple syrup.
- Lunch: Tomato and white bean salad with a side of whole-grain bread.
- Dinner: Grilled shrimp with citrus marinade, roasted asparagus, and brown rice.

Day 19:

- Breakfast: Yogurt and fruit smoothie with berries and almonds.
- Lunch: Chickpea and vegetable salad with a light vinaigrette dressing.

- Dinner: Baked chicken thighs with rosemary-garlic seasoning, roasted zucchini, and brown rice.

Day 20:

- Breakfast: Cottage cheese and mixed fruit with sunflower seeds.
- Lunch: Spinach and white bean salad with lemon vinaigrette.
- Dinner: Stir-fried lean beef with mixed vegetables and brown rice.

Day 21:

- Breakfast: Omelet with tomatoes, mushrooms, and low-fat cheese, served with whole-grain toast.
- Lunch: Red lentil and vegetable curry with a side of quinoa.
- Dinner: Grilled shrimp with a teriyaki glaze, served with steamed asparagus and wild rice.

Day 22:

- Breakfast: Yogurt and fruit smoothie with mixed berries and almonds.
- Lunch: Chickpea and vegetable salad with a light vinaigrette dressing.

- Dinner: Baked chicken thighs with rosemary-garlic seasoning, roasted zucchini, and brown rice.

Day 23:

- Breakfast: Cottage cheese and mixed fruit with sunflower seeds.
- Lunch: Spinach and white bean salad with lemon vinaigrette.
- Dinner: Stir-fried lean beef with mixed vegetables and brown rice.

Day 24:

- Breakfast: Omelet with tomatoes, mushrooms, and low-fat cheese, served with whole-grain toast.
- Lunch: Red lentil and vegetable curry with a side of quinoa.
- Dinner: Grilled shrimp with a teriyaki glaze, served with steamed asparagus and wild rice.

Day 25:

- Breakfast: Cottage cheese and mixed fruit with sunflower seeds.
- Lunch: Spinach and white bean salad with lemon vinaigrette.

- Dinner: Stir-fried lean beef with mixed vegetables and brown rice.

Day 26:

- Breakfast: Yogurt and fruit smoothie with mixed berries and almonds.
- Lunch: Chickpea and vegetable salad with a light vinaigrette dressing.
- Dinner: Baked chicken thighs with rosemary-garlic seasoning, roasted zucchini, and brown rice.

Day 27:

- Breakfast: Omelet with tomatoes, mushrooms, and low-fat cheese, served with whole-grain toast.
- Lunch: Red lentil and vegetable curry with a side of quinoa.
- Dinner: Grilled shrimp with a teriyaki glaze, served with steamed asparagus and wild rice.

Day 28:

- Breakfast: Cottage cheese and mixed fruit with sunflower seeds.
- Lunch: Spinach and white bean salad with lemon vinaigrette.

- Dinner: Stir-fried lean beef with mixed vegetables and brown rice.

Day 29:

- Breakfast: Yogurt and fruit smoothie with mixed berries and almonds.
- Lunch: Chickpea and vegetable salad with a light vinaigrette dressing.
- Dinner: Baked chicken thighs with rosemary-garlic seasoning, roasted zucchini, and brown rice.

Day 30:

- Breakfast: Omelet with tomatoes, mushrooms, and low-fat cheese, served with whole-grain toast.
- Lunch: Red lentil and vegetable curry with a side of quinoa.
- Dinner: Grilled shrimp with a teriyaki glaze, served with steamed asparagus and wild rice.

Kidney-Friendly Recipes for Seniors with Stage 3 Kidney Disease

Baked Chicken with Herbs and Quinoa

Ingredients:

- 1 skinless, boneless chicken breast
- 1 tablespoon of olive oil
- 1 teaspoon of mixed dried herbs (rosemary, thyme, or oregano)
- 1/2 cup of cooked quinoa

Directions:

- Preheat the oven to 375 degrees Fahrenheit (190 degrees Celsius).
- Brush the chicken breast with olive oil and season with herbs.
- Bake for 30 to 35 minutes, or until the chicken is cooked through.
- Serve with cooked quinoa on the side.

Portion Size: 1 serving

Nutritional Information:

- Calories: 301

- Carbohydrates: 22g
- Protein: 34g
- Fat: 11g
- Fiber: 4g
- Potassium: 353mg
- Sodium: 103mg
- Phosphorus: 254mg

Scrambled Eggs with Spinach and Tomatoes

Ingredients:

- 2 large eggs
- 1 cup of fresh spinach
- 1/2 cup of diced tomatoes
- 1 teaspoon of olive oil

Directions:

- In a nonstick skillet over medium heat, heat the olive oil.
- Sauté the spinach and diced tomatoes for 2-3 minutes.
- In a bowl, whisk the eggs and pour them over the cooked veggies, stirring constantly until thoroughly cooked.

Portion Size: 1 serving

Nutritional Information:

- Calories: 221
- Carbohydrates: 12g
- Protein: 14g
- Fat: 13g
- Fiber: 4g
- Potassium: 306mg
- Sodium: 155mg
- Phosphorus: 209mg

Grilled Shrimp Salad with Balsamic Vinaigrette

Ingredients:

- 1 cup of grilled shrimp
- 2 cups of mixed greens (lettuce, spinach, arugula)
- 1/4 cup of cherry tomatoes, halved
- 2 tablespoons of balsamic vinaigrette

Directions:

- On a platter, arrange mixed greens and cherry tomatoes.
- Drizzle with balsamic vinaigrette and top with grilled shrimp.

Portion Size: 1 serving

Nutritional Information:

- Calories: 190
- Carbohydrates: 12g
- Protein: 22g
- Fat: 9g
- Fiber: 5g
- Potassium: 255mg
- Sodium: 204mg
- Phosphorus: 153mg

Recipe: Baked Salmon with Lemon and Dill

Ingredients:

- 1 salmon fillet
- 1 tablespoon of lemon juice
- 1 teaspoon of dried dill

Directions:

- Preheat the oven to 375 degrees Fahrenheit (190 degrees Celsius).
- Line a baking sheet with parchment paper and place the salmon fillet on it.
- Sprinkle with dried dill and drizzle with lemon juice.
- Bake the fish for 12-15 minutes, or until flaky.

Portion Size: 1 serving

Nutritional Information:

- Calories: 202
- Carbohydrates: 0g
- Protein: 26g
- Fat: 9g
- Fiber: 0g
- Potassium: 310mg
- Sodium: 120mg
- Phosphorus: 203mg

Mixed Fruit Salad with Greek Yogurt

Ingredients:

- 1 cup of mixed fruits (strawberries, blueberries, and sliced peaches)
- 1/2 cup of Greek yogurt
- 1 tablespoon of honey

Directions:

In a mixing dish, combine the mixed fruits.

With a dollop of Greek yogurt and a sprinkle of honey, serve.

Portion Size: 1 serving

Nutritional Information:

- Calories: 152
- Carbohydrates: 32g
- Protein: 6g
- Fat: 3g
- Fiber: 6g
- Potassium: 253mg
- Sodium: 53mg
- Phosphorus: 152mg

Chickpea Salad with Lemon-Tahini Dressing

Ingredients:

- 1 cup of canned chickpeas
- 1/2 cup of diced cucumbers
- 1/4 cup of diced bell peppers
- 2 tablespoons of lemon-tahini dressing

Directions:

- In a mixing basin, combine chickpeas, cucumbers, and bell peppers.
- Toss gently with the lemon-tahini dressing.

Portion Size: 1 serving

Nutritional Information:

- Calories: 206
- Carbohydrates: 32g
- Protein: 11g
- Fat: 7g
- Fiber: 9g
- Potassium: 351mg
- Sodium: 124mg
- Phosphorus: 224mg

Tofu Stir-Fry with Broccoli and Brown Rice

Ingredients:

- 1 cup of cubed tofu
- 1 cup of broccoli florets
- 1 cup of cooked brown rice
- 2 tablespoons of low-sodium soy sauce

Directions:

- In a nonstick skillet over medium heat, sauté the tofu and broccoli.
- Cook for another 2-3 minutes after adding the low-sodium soy sauce.
- Serve with cooked brown rice on the side.

Portion Size: 1 serving

Nutritional Information:

- Calories: 252
- Carbohydrates: 37g
- Protein: 18g
- Fat: 6g
- Fiber: 8g
- Potassium: 352mg
- Sodium: 210mg
- Phosphorus: 255mg

Mango Cottage Cheese Bowl with Sunflower Seeds

Ingredients:

- 1/2 cup of low-fat cottage cheese
- 1/2 cup of diced mango
- 1 tablespoon of sunflower seeds

Directions:

- In a bowl, mix cottage cheese and chopped mango.
- After that, top with sunflower seeds and serve.

Portion Size: 1 serving

Nutritional Information:

- Calories: 200
- Carbohydrates: 27g

- Protein: 12g
- Fat: 8g
- Fiber: 4g
- Potassium: 305mg
- Sodium: 153mg
- Phosphorus: 202mg

Barley and Vegetable Soup with Whole-Grain Bread

Ingredients:

- 1 cup of cooked barley
- 4 cups of low-sodium vegetable broth
- 1 cup of diced mixed vegetables (carrots, celery, zucchini)
- 1 slice of whole-grain bread

Directions:

- Diced veggies, vegetable broth, and cooked barley should all be combined in a big saucepan.
- Until the veggies are soft, simmer them.
- Serve with a whole-grain bread piece on the side.

Portion Size: 1 serving

Nutritional Information:

- Calories: 222
- Carbohydrates: 45g
- Protein: 12g
- Fat: 4g
- Fiber: 12g
- Potassium: 303mg
- Sodium: 155mg
- Phosphorus: 203mg

Grilled Turkey Breast with Roasted Sweet Potatoes

Ingredients:

- 1 turkey breast slice
- 1 tablespoon of olive oil
- 1 teaspoon of dried herbs (sage, thyme, or parsley)
- 1 cup of roasted sweet potatoes

Directions:

- Preheat the grill to medium heat.
- Rub the turkey breast with olive oil and dried herbs. Grill for 6-7 minutes on each side or until fully cooked.
- Serve with a side of roasted sweet potatoes.

Portion Size: 1 serving

Nutritional Information:

- Calories: 310
- Carbohydrates: 35g
- Protein: 40g
- Fat: 15g
- Fiber: 7g
- Potassium: 352mg
- Sodium: 152mg
- Phosphorus: 254mg

Recipe: Quinoa Stuffed Bell Peppers

Ingredients:

- 2 large bell peppers
- 1 cup cooked quinoa
- 1/2 cup diced tomatoes
- 1/4 cup chopped parsley
- 1/4 cup low-sodium vegetable broth

Directions:

- Turn the oven on to 375°F, or 190°C.
- Slice off the bell peppers' tops, then take out the seeds.
- Combine chopped parsley, diced tomatoes, and cooked quinoa in a bowl.
- After packing the quinoa mixture into the bell peppers, put them in a baking dish.

- After covering the filled peppers with the vegetable broth, bake for 25 to 30 minutes.

Portion Size: 1 serving

Nutritional Information:

- Calories: 210
- Carbohydrates: 33g
- Protein: 9g
- Fat: 5g
- Fiber: 7g
- Potassium: 330mg
- Sodium: 110mg
- Phosphorus: 152mg

Apple and Walnut Chicken Salad

Ingredients:

- 1 cup cooked and diced chicken breast
- 1 small apple, diced
- 1/4 cup chopped walnuts
- 2 tablespoons plain Greek yogurt

Directions:

- Diced apple, chopped walnuts, and diced chicken breast should all be combined in a bowl.
- Greek yogurt should be added and well mixed.

Portion Size: 1 serving

Nutritional Information:

- Calories: 252
- Carbohydrates: 16g
- Protein: 22g
- Fat: 12g
- Fiber: 4g
- Potassium: 308mg
- Sodium: 155mg
- Phosphorus: 208mg

Lemon Garlic Shrimp Skewers

Ingredients:

- 1 cup large shrimp, deveined
- 1 tablespoon olive oil
- 1 clove garlic, minced
- 1 tablespoon lemon juice

Directions:

- Shrimp, lemon juice, olive oil, and minced garlic should all be combined in a bowl.
- After skewering the shrimp, grill them for two to three minutes on each side, or until they are cooked through.

Portion Size: 1 serving

Nutritional Information:

- Calories: 155
- Carbohydrates: 7g
- Protein: 22g
- Fat: 7g
- Fiber: 0g
- Potassium: 208mg
- Sodium: 103mg
- Phosphorus: 152mg

Mixed Berry Smoothie Bowl

Ingredients:

- 1 cup mixed berries (strawberries, blueberries, and raspberries)
- 1/2 cup unsweetened almond milk
- 1 tablespoon chia seeds
- 1 tablespoon sliced almonds

Directions:

- Smoothly combine almond milk and assorted fruit in a blender.
- Transfer the smoothie to a bowl and garnish with almond slices and chia seeds.

Portion Size: 1 serving

Nutritional Information:

- Calories: 211
- Carbohydrates: 27g
- Protein: 9g
- Fat: 13g
- Fiber: 9g
- Potassium: 254mg
- Sodium: 57mg
- Phosphorus: 155mg

Black Bean and Corn Salsa

Ingredients:

- 1 cup canned black beans, rinsed and drained
- 1 cup corn kernels
- 1/4 cup diced red onions
- 1/4 cup chopped cilantro
- 2 tablespoons lime juice

Directions:

- Black beans, corn kernels, chopped cilantro, and sliced red onions should all be combined in a dish.
- Pour lime juice over the blend and give it a little shake.

Portion Size: 1 serving

Nutritional Information:

- Calories: 188
- Carbohydrates: 39g
- Protein: 7g
- Fat: 5g
- Fiber: 16g
- Potassium: 309mg
- Sodium: 111mg
- Phosphorus: 215mg

Vegetable and Barley Risotto

Ingredients:

- 1 cup cooked barley
- 1 cup mixed vegetables (carrots, peas, and corn)
- 1/4 cup low-sodium vegetable broth
- 1 tablespoon grated Parmesan cheese

Directions:

- Put cooked barley, mixed veggies, and vegetable broth in a pan.
- Cook the veggies until they are soft, around medium heat.
- Before serving, top with grated Parmesan cheese.

Portion Size: 1 serving

Nutritional Information:

- Calories: 222
- Carbohydrates: 45g
- Protein: 6g
- Fat: 6g
- Fiber: 9g
- Potassium: 314mg
- Sodium: 152mg
- Phosphorus: 222mg

Grilled Tofu with Teriyaki Glaze

Ingredients:

- 1 cup tofu, pressed and sliced
- 2 tablespoons low-sodium teriyaki sauce
- 1 tablespoon sesame seeds

Directions:

- Tofu slices should be grilled for 3–4 minutes on each side over medium heat.
- When grilling, brush tofu with low-sodium teriyaki sauce.
- Before serving, top the tofu with sesame seeds.

Portion Size: 1 serving

Nutritional Information:

- Calories: 186
- Carbohydrates: 15g
- Protein: 25g
- Fat: 5g
- Fiber: 4g
- Potassium: 253mg
- Sodium: 158mg
- Phosphorus: 210mg

Roasted Vegetable Medley with Herbs

Ingredients:

- one cup of mixed veggies (zucchini, bell peppers, and onions)
- One tsp of olive oil
- One tsp of dry herb (rosemary, thyme, or oregano)

Directions:

- Set oven temperature to 400°F, or 200°C.
- Combine dry herbs and olive oil with mixed veggies.
- Bake the veggies for 20 to 25 minutes, or until they are soft.

Portion Size: 1 serving

Nutritional Information:

- Calories: 157
- Carbohydrates: 18g
- Protein: 6g
- Fat: 9g
- Fiber: 3g
- Potassium: 310mg
- Sodium: 112mg
- Phosphorus: 149mg

Poached Salmon with Dill Sauce

Ingredients:

- 1 salmon fillet
- 1/4 cup low-fat Greek yogurt
- 1 tablespoon chopped fresh dill
- 1 teaspoon lemon juice

Directions:

- Simmer the salmon fillet for 8 to 10 minutes, or until it is cooked through.
- To prepare the sauce, combine Greek yogurt, lemon juice, and chopped dill in a dish.
- Place the dill sauce over the poached fish and serve.

Portion Size: 1 serving

Nutritional Information:

- Calories: 252
- Carbohydrates: 7g
- Protein: 29g
- Fat: 15g
- Fiber: 2g
- Potassium: 354mg
- Sodium: 151mg
- Phosphorus: 245mg

Recipe: Baked Apple Chips

Ingredients:

- 1 large apple, thinly sliced
- 1 teaspoon cinnamon
- 1 tablespoon honey

Directions:

- Turn the oven on to 200°F, or 95°C.
- Toss apple slices in honey and cinnamon.
- Place apple slices on a baking sheet and bake until crispy, stirring halfway during the baking time of one to two hours.

Portion Size: 1 serving

Nutritional Information:

- Calories: 101
- Carbohydrates: 22g
- Protein: 0g
- Fat: 0g
- Fiber: 7g
- Potassium: 154mg
- Sodium: 0mg
- Phosphorus: 52mg

Understanding the Glycemic Index Diet

Diet, Obesity, Diabetes, and Kidney Disease

When it comes to managing obesity, diabetes, and renal disease, dietary considerations play a crucial role. For seniors grappling with stage 3 renal disease, maintaining stable blood sugar levels while preserving overall health and well-being is a common challenge. However, a practical and effective approach can be achieved through a diet plan that takes into account the glycemic index.

The Glycemic Index Diet for Diabetes Management

The glycemic index (GI) diet revolves around categorizing foods based on their impact on blood sugar levels. This diet has proven to be a powerful tool in managing blood glucose levels for individuals with diabetes. Emphasizing the consumption of foods with a lower glycemic index, this diet minimizes the risk of blood sugar spikes, ensuring stable levels throughout the day.

The ABCDE of Diabetes Management

The ABCDE approach to managing diabetes addresses several critical factors pivotal to controlling the condition. "A" represents A1C levels, reflecting the average blood sugar levels over the previous few months. "B" is for blood pressure control, critical in preventing kidney issues. "C" focuses on cholesterol management, essential for reducing the risk of heart disease. "D" highlights the regular use of medication and insulin, while "E" emphasizes the role of exercise in managing diabetes. Combining the glycemic index diet with this strategy can further enhance the effectiveness of diabetes management overall.

- **A: A1C Levels:** A1C levels serve as a crucial indicator of blood sugar levels over the previous two to three months. Maintaining A1C levels within the desired range, typically below 7%, is vital for preventing complications associated with diabetes. Consistent management of A1C levels significantly reduces the risk of developing chronic conditions such as renal disease, heart disease, and nerve damage.

- **B: Blood Pressure Control:** Controlling blood pressure is vital, especially for seniors with stage 3 renal disease. Elevated blood pressure can worsen the progression of renal disease and increase the risk of cardiovascular problems. Keeping blood pressure within the recommended range, typically below 130/80 mmHg, significantly reduces the risk of heart attacks, strokes, and other diabetes-related issues. Adherence to prescribed medication regimens, lifestyle adjustments, and regular monitoring are key to maintaining optimal blood pressure levels.

- **C: Cholesterol Management:** Individuals with diabetes are at an increased risk of cardiovascular complications, making cholesterol management critical. Monitoring levels of high-density lipoprotein (HDL) and low-density lipoprotein (LDL) cholesterol is essential. Controlling LDL cholesterol levels by minimizing saturated and trans fats in the diet helps reduce the risk of plaque formation in the arteries. Promoting higher levels of HDL cholesterol through regular exercise and the consumption of healthy fats further supports heart health and overall well-being.

- **D: Regular Use of Medication and Insulin:** Consistent adherence to prescribed medication and insulin regimens is crucial for effective diabetes management. Following healthcare providers' instructions for medication administration helps regulate blood sugar levels and reduces the risk of complications from uncontrolled diabetes. Proper insulin use, following recommended dosages and timings, is essential for maintaining stable blood sugar levels throughout the day. Sticking to a disciplined medication and insulin schedule, combined with regular check-ups, significantly improves overall health outcomes and disease management.

- **E: Exercise:** Regular physical exercise is a cornerstone of diabetes management and overall well-being. Exercise enhances insulin sensitivity, enabling the body to use glucose more efficiently for energy. Activities like swimming, cycling, and brisk walking can help lower blood sugar levels, reduce the risk of heart disease, and improve cardiovascular health. Incorporating exercise into daily life, as advised by healthcare professionals, is crucial for maintaining a healthy weight, managing blood sugar levels, and improving overall health.

Low Glycemic Index: Grains

Incorporating grains with a low glycemic index into the diet helps maintain stable blood sugar levels. Opting for whole grains over refined ones is advisable. Whole grains like barley, bulgur, and quinoa have a lesser impact on blood sugar. These grains contribute to improved blood sugar regulation and overall health by providing essential minerals, dietary fiber, and complex carbohydrates.

Low Glycemic Index: Vegetables

Certain vegetables, with their lower glycemic index, are more suitable for individuals with diabetes and renal disease. Non-starchy vegetables like leafy greens, broccoli, and cauliflower have a minimal effect on blood sugar levels. Rich in vitamins, minerals, and dietary fiber, these vegetables promote better glycemic control and overall health.

Low Glycemic Index: Dairy Products

Opting for dairy products with a low glycemic index aids in better blood sugar control. Choosing low-fat alternatives like skim milk and plain yogurt over full-fat dairy products minimizes their impact on blood glucose levels. These dairy options contribute to improved glucose management and provide essential minerals like calcium and vitamin D, supporting bone health.

Low Glycemic Index: Fruits

While fruits contain natural sugars, certain fruits with a lower glycemic index are more suitable for individuals with diabetes and kidney disease. Incorporating fruits with a relatively lighter impact on blood sugar levels, such as apples, berries, and cherries, helps in better glucose management. These fruits provide a range of health benefits by offering essential vitamins, minerals, and antioxidants.

Exploring Essential Nutrients and Their Sources

Understanding vital nutrients and their sources is critical in the context of controlling renal disease in seniors at stage 3. A well-balanced diet that meets particular nutritional demands while taking into account the limits imposed by the disease may considerably enhance health and well-being. Let's look at the key nutrients, where they can be found, and how they may be introduced into the diet to help seniors with stage 3 renal disease.

Protein Choices for Stage 3 Kidney Disease

Proteins are essential for muscle mass maintenance and supporting diverse body activities. Individuals with stage 3 renal disease, on the other hand, must be aware of the kind and quantity of protein taken. High-quality protein sources suited for those with impaired renal function include:

Fish: Salmon, trout, and herring are high-quality protein and omega-3 fatty acid sources that help heart health and general well-being. Grilling, roasting, or broiling salmon may help it preserve its nutritional content while reducing the amount of fat added.

Egg whites are a low-phosphorus protein that may be included in the diet of seniors with stage 3 renal disease. They supply important amino acids without the phosphorus level of the egg, making them an excellent alternative for ensuring appropriate protein consumption.

Skinless Poultry: Skinless chicken and turkey are lean protein sources that may be used in a renal diet. Grilled, baked, or roasted preparations are advised to reduce additional fat and salt consumption.

Tofu: Tofu is a low-phosphorus plant-based protein that may be incorporated into the diet of seniors with renal disease. It may be used in a variety of meals and cooked in a variety of ways to improve taste and texture.

Lean Meat Cuts: Lean cuts of beef, hog, and lamb may be eaten in moderation if they are free of visible fat. Portion control and healthier cooking techniques, such as grilling or baking, may help regulate protein intake while reducing phosphorus and salt consumption.

Protein consumption must be balanced with other dietary limitations for seniors with stage 3 renal disease. Incorporating these protein sources with caution may help preserve muscle mass and improve general health while controlling renal disease development.

Sodium and Potassium Intake Management for Seniors

Sodium and potassium are electrolytes that help the body maintain fluid equilibrium, neuron function, and muscle contractions. Individuals with stage 3 renal disease, on the other hand, must carefully monitor their salt and potassium intake to avoid fluid retention, electrolyte imbalances, and other consequences. Here are some dietary methods for regulating salt and potassium consumption in seniors with renal disease:

Limit Processed and packaged foods, such as canned soups, pre-packaged snacks, and frozen dinners, can contain excessive levels of salt. Choosing fresh, complete foods and making meals at home offers better salt management.

Pick fresh fruits and vegetables. Wisely: While all fruits and vegetables are healthful, some have a greater potassium concentration than others. Seniors with stage 3 renal disease should exercise caution while eating potassium-rich foods including bananas, oranges, and dried fruits. Lower-potassium options such as apples, berries, and peaches may aid with potassium management.

Understanding how to read food labels for salt and potassium amounts is critical for making educated decisions. Choosing

106

items with reduced salt and potassium content may help with improved electrolyte regulation in the diet.

Flavor with Herbs and Spices: Instead of depending on salt for flavor, herbs, spices, and citrus juices may improve the taste of foods without adding excessive sodium. Experimenting with various spices may provide variety and depth to meals while controlling salt consumption.

Be Wary of Condiments: Soy sauce, ketchup, and salad dressings may all be rich in salt. Using low-sodium or salt-free alternatives in moderation may help control sodium consumption while adding taste to meals.

Seniors with stage 3 renal disease must carefully regulate their salt and potassium consumption. Individuals may maintain electrolyte balance and improve overall kidney health by adding these measures to their eating regimen.

Understanding Dietary Phosphorus and Calcium Balance

Maintaining phosphorus-calcium balance is critical for seniors with stage 3 renal disease. Disruptions in this equilibrium may result in a variety of problems, including bone abnormalities and increased cardiovascular risk. Understanding the sources of phosphorus and calcium, as well as their interactions in the body, may assist seniors in efficiently managing their nutritional consumption. Here's how you get a good balance of phosphorus and calcium:

High-Phosphorus Foods Should Be Avoided: Seniors with renal disease should avoid high-phosphorus foods such as dairy products, whole grains, nuts, and some meats. Low-phosphorus substitutes, such as rice milk, cream cheese, and rice grains, may help keep phosphorus levels below the acceptable range.

Select Low-Phosphorus Dairy Substitutes: Dairy products are often rich in phosphorus. Low-phosphorus alternatives, such as almond milk, rice milk, and nondairy creamers, may deliver essential nutrients without dramatically boosting phosphorus levels in the body.

Consume Calcium-Rich Foods With Caution: While calcium is necessary for bone health, seniors with stage 3 renal disease must consume calcium-rich foods in moderation. Choosing lower-phosphorus calcium sources like cabbage, kale, and turnip greens will help maintain a healthy calcium-phosphorus balance.

Consider Phosphorus Binders: Phosphorus binders are drugs that aid in the reduction of phosphorus absorption from meals in the digestive system. Including these binders in the diet as directed by a healthcare expert may help seniors with renal disease maintain their phosphorus levels.

Keep an eye on the calcium and phosphorus ratios: Maintaining a healthy calcium-phosphorus ratio is critical for bone health. Consulting with a healthcare physician or a certified dietitian to identify the proper ratio based on individual requirements helps ensure that calcium and phosphorus levels are managed optimally.

To avoid difficulties and preserve bone health, seniors with stage 3 renal disease must balance their phosphorus and calcium consumption. Individuals may successfully regulate their dietary phosphorus and calcium intake by integrating these measures and consulting with healthcare specialists regularly.

Meal Preparation and Cooking Tips

Meal preparation and cooking skills play an important part in delivering a tasty but kidney-friendly diet for seniors in the process of treating renal disease via dietary treatments. Seniors may retain a healthy and joyful culinary experience by using appropriate cooking techniques, preparing appealing meals within dietary limitations, and skillfully organizing social events. Let's look at some crucial meal preparation and cooking recommendations for seniors with stage 3 renal disease.

Kidney-Friendly Cooking Techniques for Seniors

When it comes to cooking for seniors with stage 3 renal disease, it is critical to use kidney-friendly cooking procedures to retain nutritional content while reducing the consumption of hazardous compounds. Here are some culinary methods that are advised to meet the nutritional demands of seniors with renal disease:

- Grilling: Grilling imparts smokey characteristics to meats, seafood, and vegetables without the need for extra fats or spices. Grilled foods may be seasoned with herbs and spices to improve their flavor without dramatically increasing salt or potassium levels.

- Baking is a healthy and easy cooking method that allows for the production of a variety of foods without the need for additional oils or fats. Seniors may make delectable and kidney-friendly meals by baking lean meats, fish, and vegetables seasoned with low-sodium herbs.

- Steaming is a mild cooking technique that maintains foods' inherent tastes and minerals. Seniors may steam vegetables, fish, and chicken to keep texture and nutritional content while reducing the need for additional fats or spices.

- Boiling: Boiling is a good way to prepare grains, legumes, and vegetables without using any oils or fats. It softens food while keeping its inherent tastes, making it a good choice for seniors who want to prepare nutrient-rich and kidney-friendly meals.

- Sautéing with little Oil: Sautéing with little oil allows for the production of delectable foods while avoiding the addition of unnecessary fats. Using heart-healthy oils in moderation, such as olive oil and canola oil, may assist seniors in creating tasty and kidney-friendly meals while preserving their overall health.

111

Creating Delicious Meals While Following Dietary Restrictions:

While following dietary limitations is critical for treating renal illness, preparing enjoyable meals may be difficult at times. Seniors, with the appropriate strategy and ingredient selection, may have tasty and fulfilling meals while adhering to their dietary limitations. Here are some ideas for preparing tasty meals that are customized to the requirements of seniors with renal disease:

- Fresh herbs and spices such as basil, oregano, cilantro, and garlic may give depth and scent to dishes without the need for excessive salt or sodium-based seasonings. Experimenting with various herb and spice combinations may improve the taste and attractiveness of foods.

- Choose Citrus Juices: Citrus juices like lemon, lime, and orange may provide a tart and refreshing taste to a variety of recipes. Citrus juices may be used as natural flavor enhancers, reducing the need for salt and sodium-based seasonings and enabling seniors to enjoy meals that are both pleasant and kidney-friendly.

- Investigate Low-Sodium Condiments: Using low-sodium condiments like low-sodium soy sauce, vinegar, and spicy sauce may add taste to dishes

112

without drastically boosting salt levels. These condiments may be used sparingly to improve the flavor of foods while sticking to the dietary limitations of seniors with renal disease.

- Experiment with Low-Potassium Foods: Low-potassium items like apples, berries, and cucumbers may provide a fresh and tasty edge to meals. By including these items in salads, smoothies, and side dishes, seniors may enjoy a diversified culinary experience while properly regulating their potassium consumption.

- Make Your Stocks and Broths: Making your stocks and broths from low-sodium items may provide a tasty basis for soups, stews, and sauces. Homemade stocks and broths may be flavored with a variety of herbs and spices, enabling seniors to easily enjoy gourmet and kidney-friendly meals.

Tips for Dining Out and Managing Social Gatherings:

While dietary changes are critical for treating renal disease, seniors with stage 3 kidney disease may have difficulties while dining out or attending social events. Seniors, on the other hand, may handle these circumstances well while sticking to their dietary needs with proper planning and preparation. Here are some useful hints for eating out and socializing:

- Research Restaurant Menus in Advance: When eating out, seniors may find kidney-friendly alternatives and make educated decisions by researching restaurant menus in advance. Choosing grilled or baked foods, asking for dressings and sauces on the side, and selecting low-sodium options may all help to guarantee a pleasant eating experience while sticking to dietary restrictions.

- Communicate Dietary Needs to the Server: Communicating dietary needs to the server may assist seniors in efficiently communicating their requirements and preferences. Requesting recipe changes, and low-sodium options, and enquiring about ingredient replacements may help seniors enjoy a kidney-friendly dinner without sacrificing taste or flavor.

- Plan Potluck Contributions Carefully: When attending social gatherings or potluck events, seniors may display their culinary abilities while sticking to their dietary restrictions by preparing potluck contributions carefully. Bringing kidney-friendly items like salads, grilled veggies, and lean protein alternatives helps ensure that elders have appropriate eating selections while socializing.

- be Hydrated with Water: Seniors with stage 3 renal disease must be hydrated with water at all times, particularly while eating out or attending social events. Choosing water over sugary or alcoholic beverages may help seniors stay hydrated and promote overall renal function during the event.

- Communicate with Hosts and Peers: Openly discussing dietary limitations and preferences with hosts and peers helps encourage understanding and support in social situations. Sharing particular dietary requirements, reviewing ingredient possibilities, and volunteering to contribute kidney-friendly recipes may help seniors with stage 3 renal disease build a collaborative and inclusive atmosphere.

Lifestyle Adjustments for Seniors with Kidney Disease

When diagnosed with kidney disease, adapting to a new lifestyle is critical to properly treating the illness. Various lifestyle changes may considerably improve the general well-being and quality of life of seniors with renal disease. Seniors may manage their kidney disease journey more efficiently while keeping a positive and holistic attitude to their health by emphasizing exercise and physical activity, managing medicines and treatment regimens, and addressing emotional and mental well-being.

Incorporating Physical Activity and Exercise

Regular exercise and physical activity are important for elders with renal disease because they may improve general health, improve cardiovascular function, and promote kidney function. Here are some suggested fitness and physical activity modifications for seniors with renal disease:

Walking, cycling, and swimming are examples of low-impact aerobic workouts that may help seniors maintain cardiovascular health without placing undue pressure on their joints and muscles. Incorporating these exercises into your everyday regimen will help enhance your blood circulation and general well-being.

care in Strength Training: Integrating strength training activities with care may help seniors gain muscular strength and bone health while reducing the chance of injury. Seniors may participate in strength-building activities safely and efficiently by choosing mild resistance training and utilizing suitable equipment under the supervision of a qualified practitioner.

Flexibility and balance activities, such as yoga, tai chi, and stretching routines, may assist seniors in increasing their range of motion, improving stability, and minimizing the chance of falls or accidents. Including these activities in a regular fitness plan helps improve physical mobility and general well-being.

Mind-Body Wellness Activities: Mind-body wellness activities such as meditation, deep breathing exercises, and mindfulness methods may assist seniors in managing stress, reducing anxiety, and fostering a feeling of inner peace and relaxation. Incorporating these techniques into one's daily routine may help to enhance emotional well-being and lead to a more balanced and holistic existence.

Managing Medications and Treatment Plans:

To guarantee correct symptom management, disease progression control, and overall health maintenance, seniors with kidney disease must effectively manage medicines and treatment programs. Here are some important factors to consider while managing medicines and treatment programs for elders with renal disease:

Adherence to Medication regimens: Seniors must adhere to recommended medication regimens to obtain the best treatment results and maintain stable renal function. Following a regular medication schedule as recommended by healthcare specialists may help elders manage their illness efficiently and avoid any risks linked with non-adherence.

Regular Monitoring and Follow-ups: For elders with renal disease, regular monitoring of kidney function and follow-up consultations with healthcare specialists are crucial. Routine check-ups, laboratory testing, and meetings with nephrologists or healthcare experts may give elders useful insights into their disease and assist them in making educated treatment choices.

Adjustments to Diet and Lifestyle: Including dietary and lifestyle changes as indicated by healthcare specialists may supplement medication management and treatment

118

strategies for elders with renal disease. Adhering to kidney-friendly diets, exercising regularly, and applying stress-reduction practices might help drugs work better and contribute to improved overall health results.

Understanding Potential Side Effects: Seniors with renal disease must be informed of potential side effects and adverse reactions linked with prescription drugs. Understanding the potential dangers and advantages of drugs, being alert for any odd symptoms or responses, and talking with healthcare experts as soon as possible may help seniors manage their treatment regimens more successfully and reduce the risk of problems.

Emotional and Mental Well-being Support for Seniors:

Addressing seniors' emotional and mental well-being is important because it may have a substantial influence on their quality of life, mood, and overall view of their health journey. Here are some crucial ways to assist elders with renal disease with their emotional and mental well-being:

Support Groups and Counseling: Attending support groups and counseling sessions may allow seniors to connect with others who are dealing with similar health issues, exchange experiences, and get emotional support. Participating in support groups, counseling sessions, and peer conversations may help seniors overcome feelings of loneliness and build a sense of community and understanding.

Stress Management methods: Stress management methods such as mindfulness practices, relaxation exercises, and stress-reduction measures may assist seniors in coping with the emotional weight associated with renal disease treatment. Incorporating these approaches into everyday routines may help to increase emotional resilience, coping skills, and general well-being.

Open Communication and Expressing: Promoting open communication and the expressing of sentiments and concerns may help seniors communicate their emotions, worries, and anxiety about their health journey. Creating a friendly and nonjudgmental atmosphere in which elders may express their ideas, ask questions, and seek help can promote emotional stability and encourage a proactive approach to treating mental well-being.

Participation in holistic wellness programs that incorporate diverse aspects of physical, emotional, and mental well-being may offer elders a complete approach to health management. Engaging in wellness programs that include exercise, mindfulness practices, and educational resources may help seniors with renal disease live a more holistic and balanced lifestyle.

Conclusion

As we near the end of this fascinating trip into the complexities of a renal disease diet suited for seniors in stage 3, it becomes clear that the importance of following a particular dietary plan cannot be stressed. We have dug into the many facets of kidney disease management throughout this book, highlighting the crucial role of nutrition in encouraging improved health outcomes, improving overall well-being, and creating a proactive attitude to treating this complicated illness. Let us explore the necessity of following a renal disease diet for seniors, stress the need to take a proactive approach to health and well-being, and present essential resources for more information and assistance as we reflect on the major lessons from our conversations.

Summary of the Importance of a Kidney Disease Diet for Seniors

A kidney disease diet suited for seniors in stage 3 is a cornerstone in the condition's complete therapy, playing a critical role in preserving normal kidney function, regulating related symptoms, and decreasing the risk of future consequences. Seniors may greatly improve their general health and well-being by highlighting the necessity of sticking to dietary recommendations centered on managing potassium, sodium, and phosphorus consumption. The incorporation of kidney-friendly foods, portion control tactics, and thoughtful meal planning enables seniors to take proactive steps toward improved blood pressure management, healthier renal function, and a greater quality of life. As we outline the significance of a renal disease diet, it is important to emphasize the transforming influence that dietary changes may have on seniors' health, highlighting the power of nutrition in molding their health journey and enhancing their long-term prognosis.

Promoting a Proactive Approach to Health and Wellness

Promoting a proactive approach to health and well-being is critical for seniors with renal disease, as it allows them to take control of their health journey, make educated choices, and actively engage in their treatment programs. Seniors may create a feeling of resilience, foster a positive outlook, and improve their overall quality of life by adopting proactive measures such as regular exercise, sticking to prescribed medicines, and prioritizing emotional and mental well-being. Empowering elders to advocate for their health, seek important resources and support, and create open communication with healthcare practitioners may encourage a collaborative approach to renal disease treatment and a more holistic and complete approach to health management. Seniors may manage their health journey with confidence, resilience, and a better feeling of control by cultivating a proactive mentality and establishing a sense of empowerment, eventually leading to improved health outcomes and higher well-being.

Final Thoughts and Resources for Further Information

As we near the end of our investigation into the renal disease diet for seniors on stage 3, it is critical to give excellent options for more information and assistance, allowing seniors to access comprehensive advice, educational materials, and community services to help them on their health journey. Seniors may discover a variety of knowledge, assistance, and peer support to aid their continuous health management by providing access to credible organizations, internet platforms, and support groups specialized in renal disease management. Furthermore, giving thorough lists of educational resources, credible websites, and nephrology-specific healthcare providers may enable seniors to remain informed, make intelligent choices, and seek dependable assistance as they navigate their health journey. Seniors may continue to grow their knowledge, build a feeling of community, and stay actively involved in their health management by providing access to these excellent resources, eventually leading to better health outcomes and overall well-being.

Finally, the trip through the complexities of the renal disease diet for seniors on stage 3 has shed light on the transformational power of nutrition, lifestyle changes, and proactive health management. We hope to empower seniors to embark on their health journey with confidence, resilience, and a deep sense of empowerment by recognizing the critical importance of following a specialized dietary plan, embracing a proactive approach to health and well-being, and providing valuable resources for additional information and support. May this book serve as a guide, encouraging elders to take a holistic approach to their health and well-being.